F

LISA K. WEISS

Illustrated by Victoria Roberts

A FIRESIDE BOOK
Published by Simon & Schuster
NEW YORK LONDON TORONTO SYDNEY TOKYO SINGAPORE

YOU JUST GLOW!

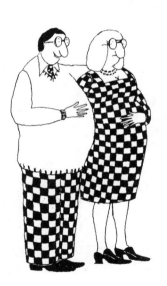

AND OTHER

LIES OF

PREGNANCY,

CHILDBIRTH,

AND BEYOND

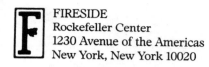

FIRESIDE
Rockefeller Center
1230 Avenue of the Americas
New York, New York 10020

FIRESIDE and colophon are registered trademarks
of Simon & Schuster Inc.

Designed by Stanley S. Drate/Folio Graphics Co. Inc.
Manufactured in the United States of America

10   9   8   7   6   5   4   3

Library of Congress Cataloging-in-Publication Data
Weiss, Lisa K.
    You just glow! : and other lies of pregnancy, childbirth, and
beyond / Lisa K. Weiss ; illustrated by Victoria Roberts.
        p.   cm.
    "A Fireside book."
    1. Pregnancy—Humor.   2. Childbirth—Humor.   I. Title.
PN6231.P68W45   1994
818'.5402—dc20   94-14851   CIP
ISBN 0-671-86969-8

ACKNOWLEDGMENTS

First, I want to thank my editors at Simon & Schuster: Sheridan Hay, for having a sense of humor and for being pregnant at the right time, and Sydny Miner, for painlessly guiding me through this process.

I want to thank Victoria Roberts for "getting it" so immediately and for translating and enhancing my words so perfectly.

I also want to acknowledge the special help and guidance so generously offered to me by my friend and attorney, Lisa Lipman.

And finally, I want to thank my husband, Michael Schwartzman, for encouraging me and for laughing in all the right places.

To my husband, Michael, who never lied to me,
To my children, Joey, Adam and Lianna, whose presence made
   all the lies not matter,
To my mother, Pearl, who *did* make a wonderful baby nurse when
   I really needed her,
To my father, Stan, who made it easy for her to come help me,
And to my doctor, David Fields, who told me the truth about
   premature labor. Twice.
—L.K.W.

For Margaret Morgan
—V.R.

INTRODUCTION

When I was little and got my first immunization, the pediatrician was honest and told me that the shots would hurt badly for a few seconds. When I was seven and learning to swim, the instructor told me frankly that until I learned the proper way to dive, I would keep getting water up my nose. When I first got braces on my teeth, the orthodontist was clear and direct; he explained that my mouth would be sore in the morning, every morning that I wore them. When I was eleven and dared to take my first puff of a cigarette, my worldly-wise best friend told me in very matter-of-fact tones that the smoke would burn my throat and make me cough. When I first got my period, the school nurse warned me not to be surprised if I got excruciating cramps every month. When I first decided to have sex, my college roommate candidly admitted to me that it would probably hurt the first time. When I got pregnant, honesty, directness, frankness, and candor took a vacation.

When I first got pregnant, everyone told me how great I looked, how lucky I was, how happy I must be. When I got desperately hungry all the time, feeling that I was going to die if I didn't get

Cantonese shrimp in lobster sauce and coffee ice cream with whipped cream *immediately*, everyone told me that it would soon pass and I'd be back to my normal, only-slightly-bingey self in no time. When I started throwing up every morning, everyone told me that it would soon pass and I'd be feeling fine in no time. When I started to get backaches and leg pains and dents in my shoulders from my heavy-duty bra straps, everyone told me that these physical discomforts would soon subside. When my husband and I took a prepared childbirth course, everyone said that breathing exercises and relaxation techniques would help immensely during labor. Everyone lied.

All through my pregnancy my husband kept telling me that we didn't need my mother to come and stay with us; we didn't need a baby nurse. He was going to take time off and stay home with me the first week to help take care of me and the baby. The next thing I knew, he just needed to go to the office for a couple of hours late in the afternoon to check on a few things. The next thing I knew, late afternoon started at ten in the morning and a couple of hours lasted until dinnertime.

Why didn't someone tell me?

PART ONE

PREGNANCY

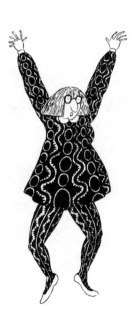

We're pregnant!

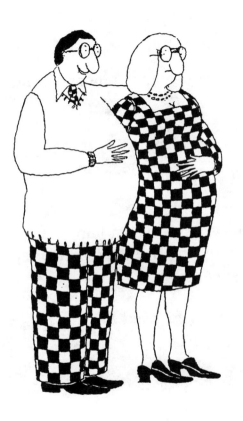

Directions for at-home pregnancy tests are simple.

～

After the baby comes, I'll arrange my hours to be home earlier.

～

Most women find they can limit their weight gain to about twenty pounds during pregnancy.

～

You'll get used to throwing up.

～

I'll help with the housework on weekends.

The second trimester will be easier.

❧

Your new, fuller figure makes you
look Rubensesque.

❧

Increasing physical activity relieves constipation.

❧

Practicing Kegel exercises regularly helps control
your bladder.

❧

Switching to low heels prevents leg cramps.

Eat a cracker before you get out of bed in the morning and you won't be nauseous.

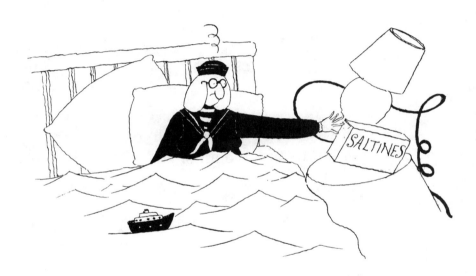

The tenderness in your breasts will diminish after the first month or so.

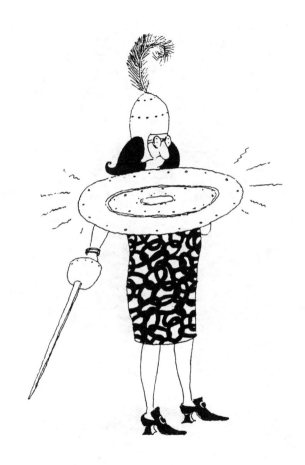

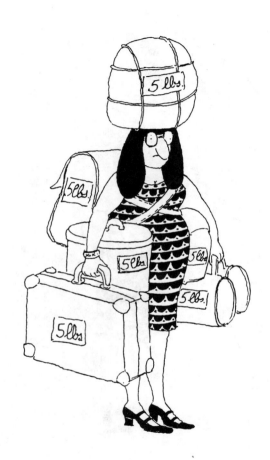

Five pounds is about all most women gain during the first trimester.

Pregnancy brings out the best in your hair, making
it full and lustrous!

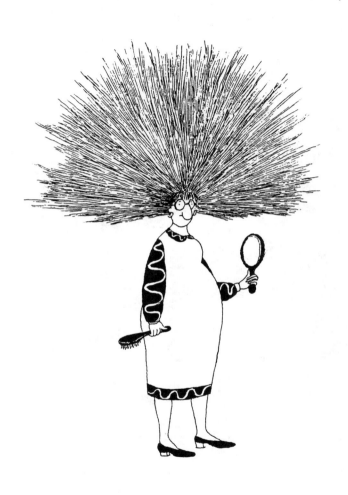

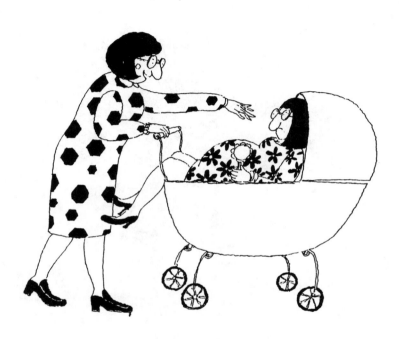

When you're pregnant, you just naturally get closer to your own mother.

When the baby turns over and kicks, it feels like little butterflies gently fluttering around.

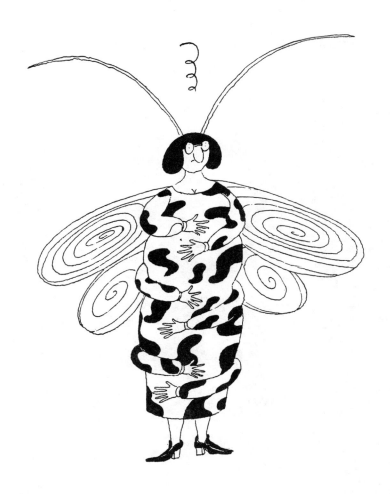

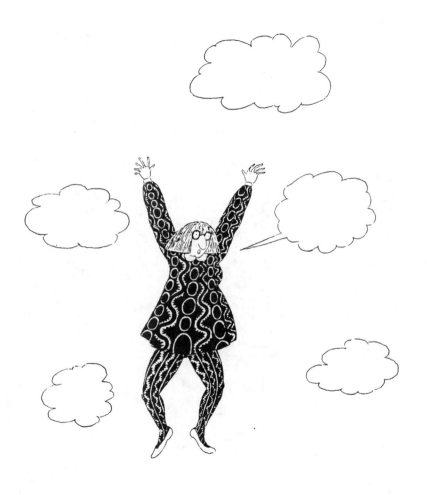

You can relieve "air hunger" by taking slow, deep breaths.

Eating slowly reduces heartburn.

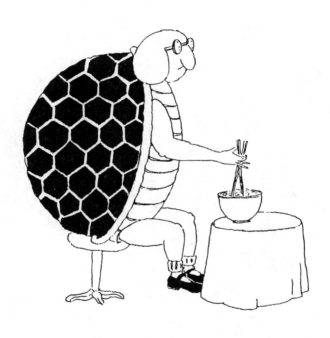

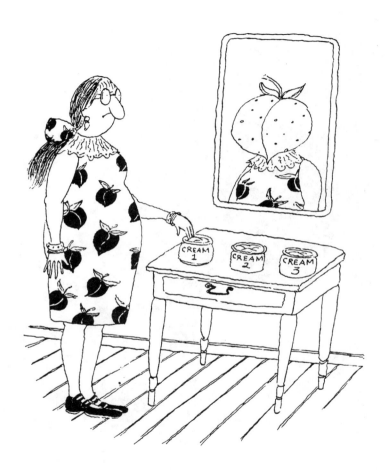

Pregnancy gives you a peaches-and-cream complexion.

Just wear a good supportive bra, and your breasts will return to their prepregnancy shape and size in no time.

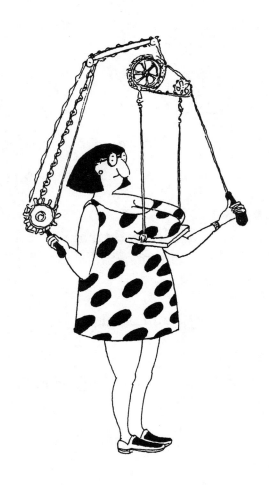

Ultrasound reliably determines your baby's sex.

❧

This amniocentesis needle won't hurt a bit.

❧

Those shoulder pads make you look
so much slimmer!

❧

You just glow!

❧

The third trimester will be easier.

Braxton-Hicks contractions feel like a little "tightening" sensation.

◆

People are so considerate of pregnant women, you'll never have trouble getting a seat on the bus.

◆

This pelvic exam won't hurt.

◆

Having your own mother as your baby nurse is a great idea!

Those vertical stripes make you look
so much slimmer!

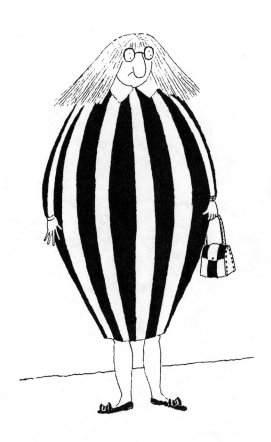

No, honey, you're even more attractive to me now
that you're carrying our child!

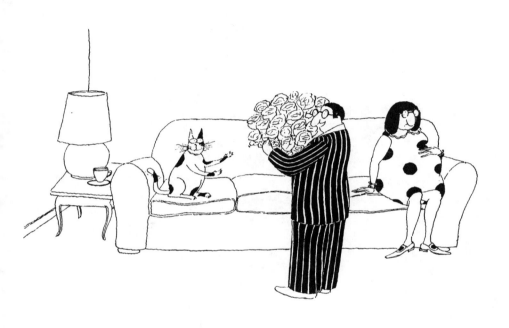

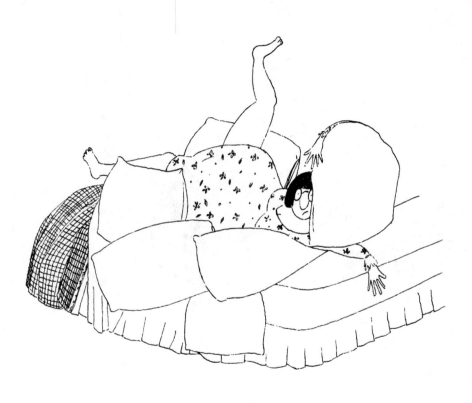

A few pillows and you'll find you sleep comfortably
in these later months.

Your boss will understand if you need to leave work
a little earlier during those last few weeks.

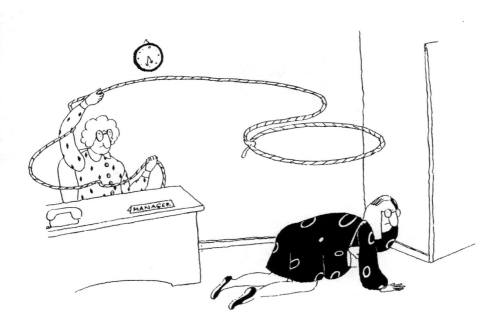

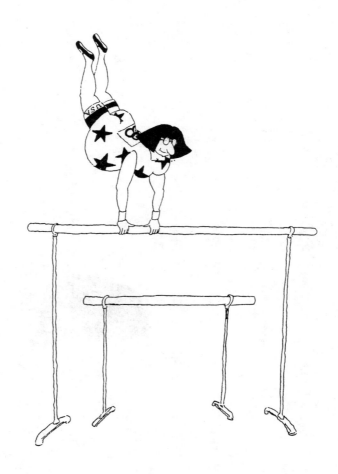

You can continue your regular exercise routine throughout your pregnancy.

You'll get an extra burst of energy in the last trimester so you can get the nursery ready—it's called "nesting."

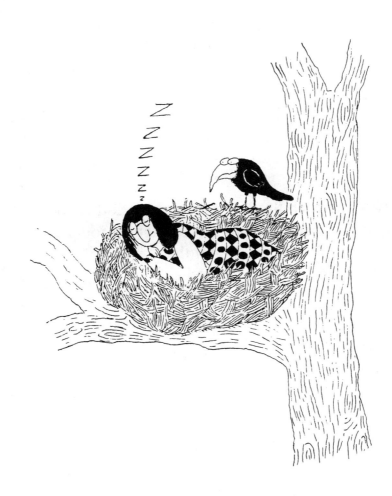

They make such flattering maternity clothes today, you can look downright stylish right through the ninth month!

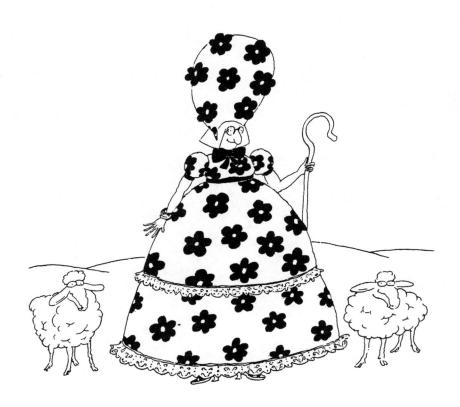

PART TWO
CHILDBIRTH

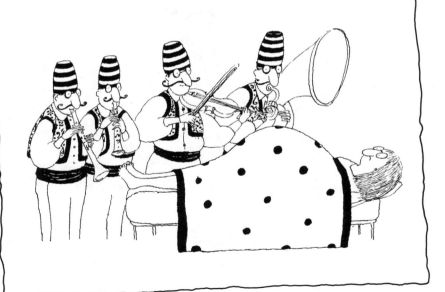

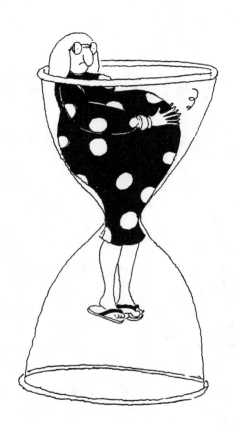

Your "due date" will accurately predict when you'll deliver.

If you exercise during the nine months, your labor will be a breeze!

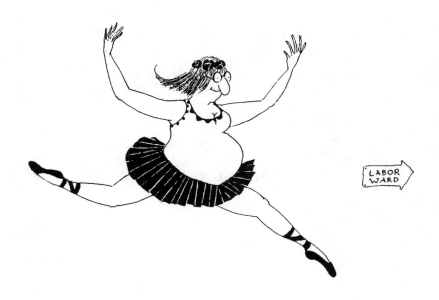

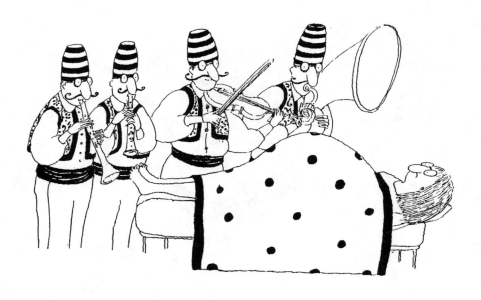

Listening to your favorite music can provide a pleasant and soothing distraction through the early stages of labor.

There are so many different kinds of effective pain medications today that there's no reason for you to be the least bit uncomfortable!

❧

Sucking on ice chips can really satisfy your thirst.

❧

The birthing room is just like home!

❧

There's nothing to worry about.

Stroking the abdomen provides valuable relief
during strong contractions.

❧

A back rub will take care of that back labor.

❧

You're doing wonderfully!

❧

When this is all over, you won't even remember
the pain.

If you breathe properly, you won't feel
the discomfort.

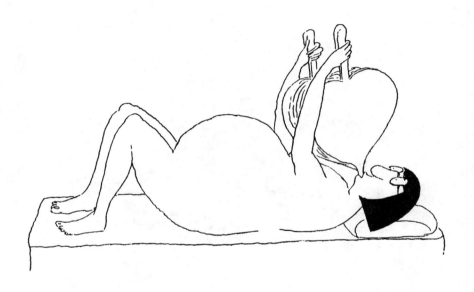

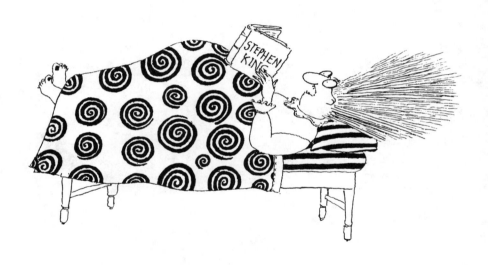

Many women find it relaxing to read a good book
between contractions.

If you use positive imagery, you'll barely notice the contractions.

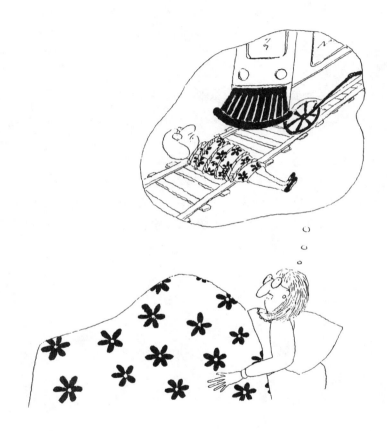

You'll be so excited, you won't even notice that you're sharing a labor room.

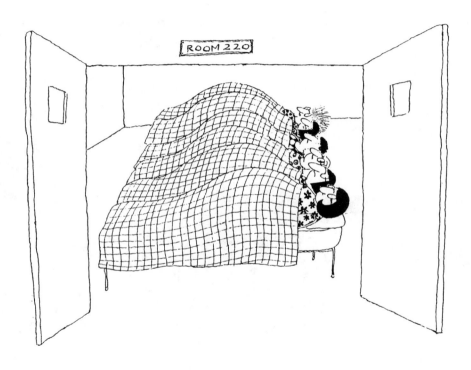

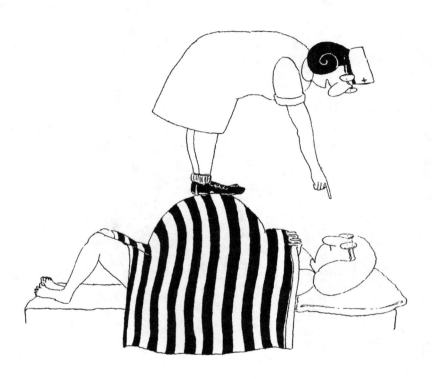

The nurses are there to make you more comfortable.

You'll be so absorbed with labor, you won't notice that you're starving.

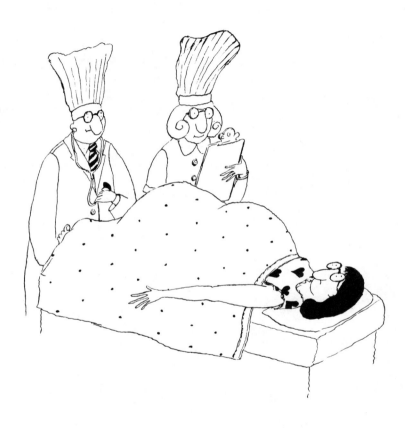

This procedure is simply routine.

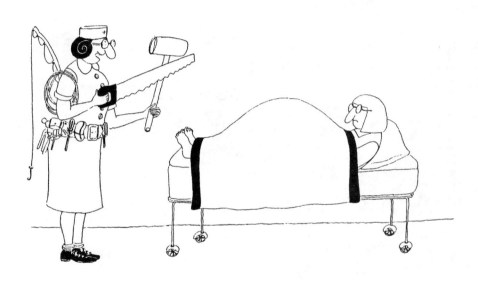

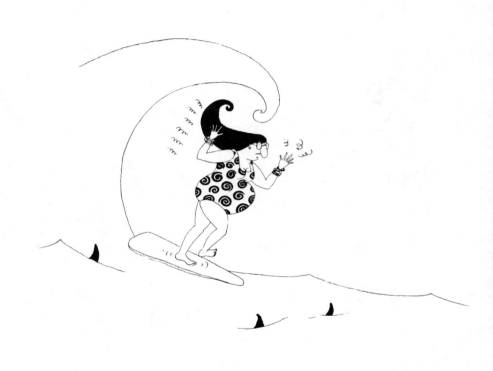

Just "go with the flow" and you'll be fine.

Changing positions during labor will make you feel more comfortable.

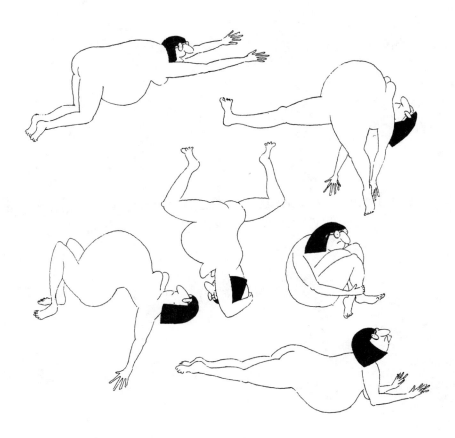

If you just concentrate on the pushing, it'll be over in a flash!

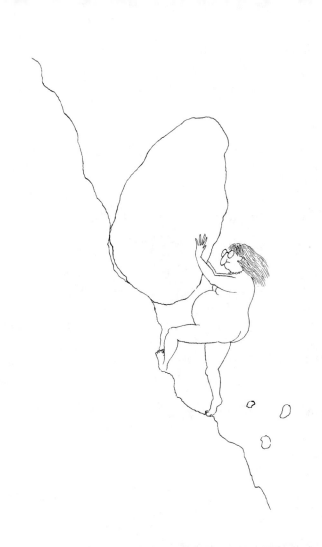

The contraction's over; you can rest now.

❧

Transfer from the labor room to the delivery room
is easy.

❧

You look beautiful!

❧

Relax, and you'll fully enjoy the wondrous miracle
of giving birth.

Hard labor only lasts for an hour or so.

❧

Just a little bit longer!

❧

You'll find the hospital a quiet and calm place to rest and recover.

❧

Once you're home, the bleeding will stop within a day or two.

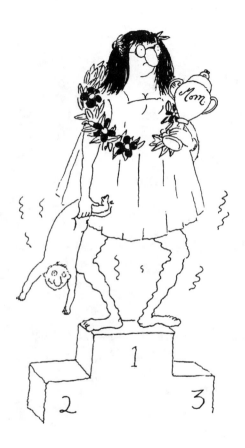

Congratulations; you did that like a pro!

After delivery, you won't even feel the doctor stitching up the episiotomy.

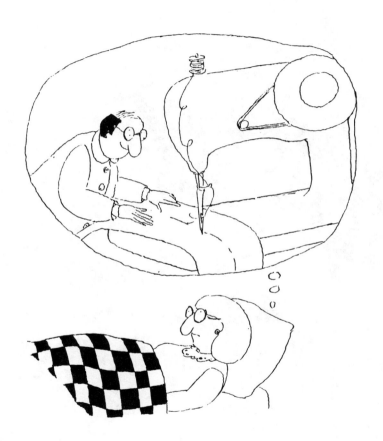

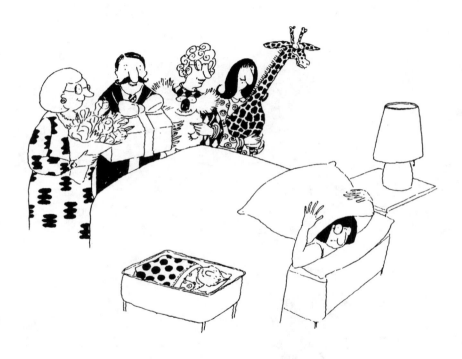

Once the baby's born, you'll enjoy having lots of visitors to share your joy.

Keep ice on your episiotomy and, by the next day, you'll barely notice it.

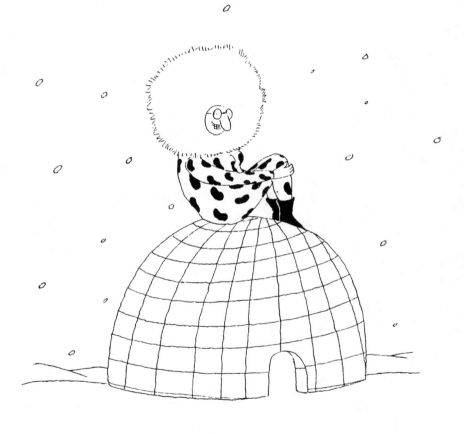

Just-born babies are so beautiful!

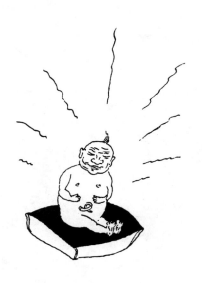

PART THREE
AND BEYOND

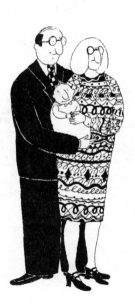

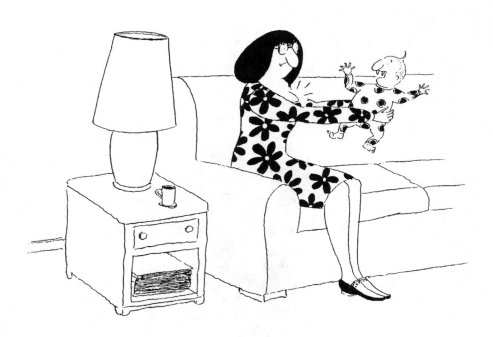

Nursing a teething baby is simple; babies don't bite.

When you come home from the hospital, everyone will understand if you need a day or two before you want visitors.

❧

He was so supportive!

❧

Nursing is such a communion with your baby—it's almost a religious experience.

❧

I'll give him the 2 A.M. bottle; I promise!

You and your baby will know instinctively
how to nurse.

❧

Warm washcloths will ease the slight discomfort you
may feel when you're engorged.

❧

Nursing makes it easier to lose the weight
you've gained.

❧

Those thigh-length tunics make you look
so much slimmer!

The "football hold" is all you need to calm
a colicky baby.

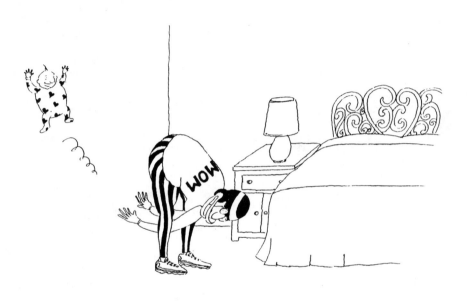

A warm bath will soothe the tension of
a colicky baby.

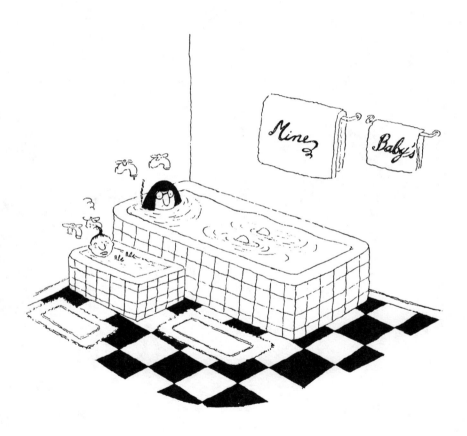

Aloe will make those stretch marks disappear.

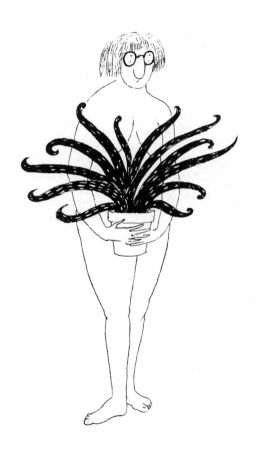

If you exercise, you'll have more energy.

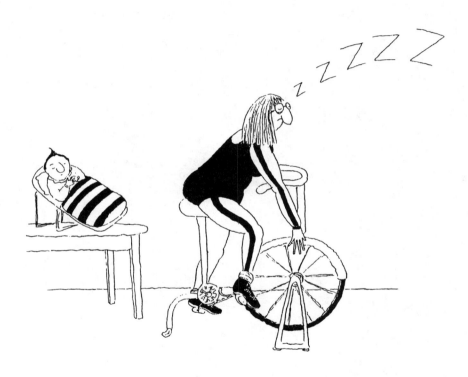

You'll get used to less sleep; you'll be surprised how you adjust!

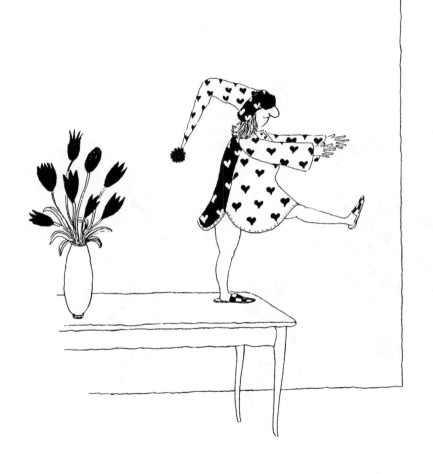

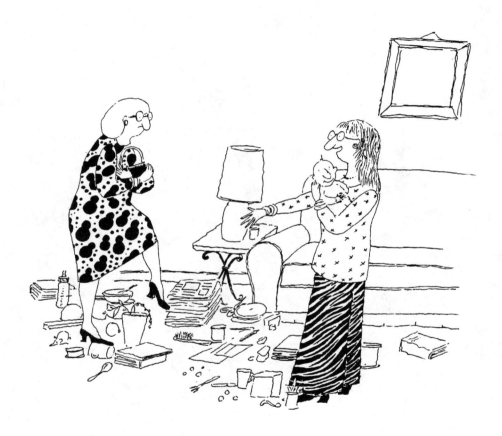

Let the housework go for a while;
guests will understand.

If you keep his room dark, he'll fall back to sleep by himself.

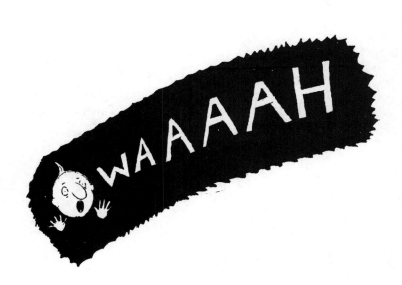

Your baby won't need to nurse more than every
three to four hours.

❧

Colic typically lasts only a week or two.

❧

It gets easier, I promise.

❧

He's just got day and night reversed; that'll right
itself in a few days.

If you just let him cry for a night or two, he'll learn to put himself to sleep.

❧

You can nap when your baby naps.

❧

That's nothing to worry about.

❧

Just develop a bedtime routine, and he'll go to sleep easier.

Weaning your child from breast to bottle is painless if you do it gradually.

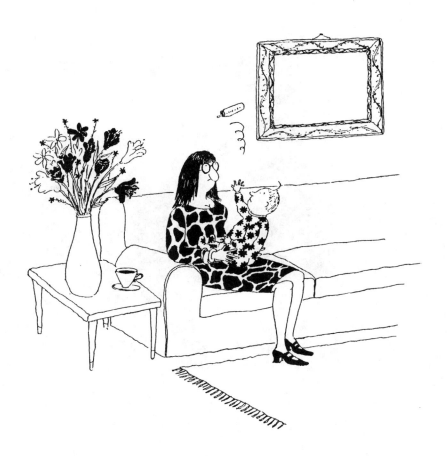

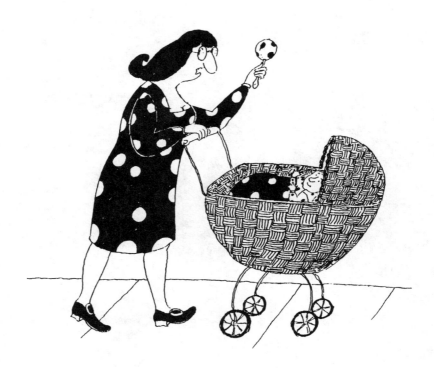

Being an older mother means you'll have
more patience.

We really share taking care of the baby fifty-fifty.

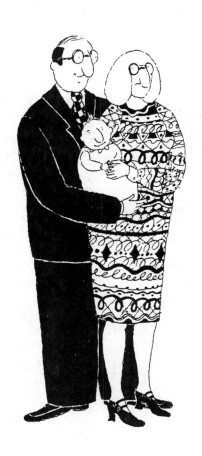

Your baby should sleep through the night
by six months.

❧

Sibling rivalry can be minimized by simply making
sure you save some "alone time" for each child.

❧

Teething doesn't cause fevers.

He can't choke on a Cheerio; it dissolves
in the mouth!

❧

When he gives up his morning nap, he won't fight
you about going to sleep at night anymore.

You can have sex again in six weeks.

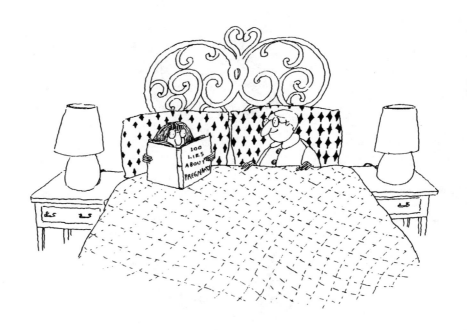

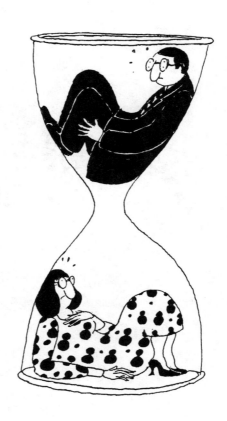

You've just got to make time for each other.

The second one will be easier.

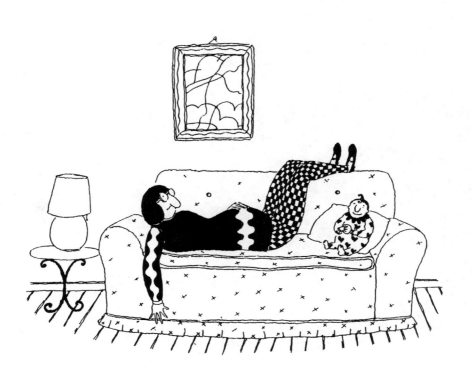